Slow Cooker

Simple Tasty Slow Cooker Recipes and Healthy and Delicious Crockpot Recipes for Beginners

Marie Getty

Published by David Kruse Publishing House

Slow Cooker: Simple Tasty Slow Cooker Recipes and Healthy and Delicious Crockpot Recipes for Beginners

ISBN 978-1-9992832-5-4

Legal & Disclaimer

The information contained in this book is not designed to replace or take the place of any form of medicine or professional medical advice. The information in this book has been provided for educational and entertainment purposes only.

The information contained in this book has been compiled from sources deemed reliable, and it is accurate to the best of the Author's knowledge; however, the Author cannot guarantee its accuracy and validity and cannot be held liable for any errors or omissions. Changes are periodically made to this book. You must consult your doctor or get professional medical advice before using any of the suggested remedies, techniques, or information in this book.

Upon using the information contained in this book, you agree to hold harmless the Author from and against any damages, costs, and expenses, including any legal fees potentially resulting from the application of any of the information provided by this guide. This disclaimer applies to any damages or injury caused by the use and application, whether directly or indirectly, of any advice or information presented, whether for breach of contract, tort, negligence, personal injury, criminal intent, or under any other cause of action.

You agree to accept all risks of using the information presented inside this book. You need to consult a professional medical practitioner in order to ensure you are both able and healthy enough to participate in this program.

TABLE OF CONTENTS

Part -1

Introduction

I want to thank you and congratulate you for downloading the book.

This book contains proven steps and strategies on how to make slow cooking simple and efficient.

Slow cooking has become very popular due to the convenience it brings to every busy family out there. Also, it's a stepping stone for those who would like to learn more about cooking and have not figured out how to start just yet.

Cooking a nice homemade meal is always better than opening and boiling artificially flavored mac and cheese. Preparing a homemade meal is healthier, easier, and much more convenient now, thanks to the wonders of slow cooking.

People are usually too busy to prepare a nice dish for themselves. Going to restaurants can be a bit upsetting to the pocket, and too much fast food will definitely send you racing to the emergency room due to a problematic health condition.

Preparing a convenient, healthy meal is just what people need. And using the slow cooker or Crock-Pot might just be the key! For those of you who have no idea how to begin or start, or maybe just clueless about how the art of slow cooking works, then please read on.

This book will give you a step-by-step guide and tips regarding slow cooking, as well as the best basic ingredients which will work well with any type of dish you would like to prepare. This will work great for those of you who are always on the go or don't have enough time to multitask and juggle chores and cooking. Learning the basics is always the best way to start.

You'll also learn some techniques to maximize the advantages of slow cooking: the best ingredients to add, tips and tricks to maximize everything in the kitchen, and easy-to-make recipes which will definitely help make your culinary experience more enjoyable and convenient.

Everything you need to know about this great cooking method is within these pages — starting with three-ingredient dishes which will work wonders for every busy person, dos and don'ts, how to maximize your budget when picking certain ingredients for your dish, and a couple of safety reminders.

Thanks again for downloading this book, I hope you enjoy it!

Chapter 1: The Benefits of Slow Cooking

Everyday life is taking its toll on every busy mom and dad out there. Whether they work their brains out at the office, or they're just simply taking care of their kids and the household chores, it's just quite impossible to find time to prepare a nice family meal due to all the things they are being demanded of.

Even those who don't have families of their own find it difficult to whip up their own homemade meal, given the demands of their job and social life.

A family dinner, despite what most people think, is very important. It promotes quality time and communication and strengthens the bond within a household which, of course, is one of the few basic things needed to create a happy and healthy home.

Slow cooking is essential in the culinary world. It provides the meal with a well-balanced taste that really captures attention. By simmering the meat and/or vegetables in slow heat, the richness and flavor of the dish is balanced, thereby creating good texture and locking in the moisture the meat needs to make the food appealing to the stomach. And the good thing about it is you can mimic this at home to your own advantage!

Slow cooking is ideal for busy people in order to buy them time to relax a bit. If you're quite busy doing things around the house, this might be what you need to provide yourself enough time to prepare a hearty meal for yourself or for the whole family and at the same time, finish all the tasks you need to do while waiting for your food to cook.

On the other hand, if you're just starting to learn how to cook, this is also the first thing you need to cover. Slow cooking doesn't have to be too complicated since you're just bringing everything to a rich boil. It works best as well for people who are not that familiar yet with cooking because you'll learn all the basics without sacrificing the quality of the dish you are making.

Making It Easier

Indeed, slow cooking is an advantage — whether it comes to preparing the family meal, buying more time to bring everything altogether, or just simply trying to learn the basic necessities of cooking. Who doesn't want enough time to try another recipe while waiting, or simply just read a good book while you wait for your ingredients to fully burst in rich flavors?

Of course, it's no use if the recipe calls for hundreds of condiments and ingredients to be added gradually to the simmering pot. It goes against the purpose or benefit of why you want to learn how to slow cook in the first place. (Although, of course, it doesn't hurt adding a bit of wonder to what you're cooking.) If a quick and simple meal guide is what you are really looking for then, you can make everything easier by just adding three basic ingredients altogether.

Combining three basic ingredients is the perfect solution to those who don't quite know yet what ingredients will work best with slow cooking, or those who just can't be bothered to do a lot of work in the kitchen.

Also, slow cooking benefits those who simply just cannot find enough time to go back and forth to check on or add other things to the simmering pot. The following chapters will give you some easy ideal recipes which include only three ingredients for slow cooking — what's more, you can improvise these recipes in the future in order to help create a suitable meal that everyone can enjoy.

Chapter 2: The Best Tools To Use For Slow Cooking

What would you first consider before putting everything together?

The answer is simple: a Crock-Pot or a slow cooker.

It's important to know the difference between the two for you to know what will work best with what you're whipping up. If you have enough knowledge to distinguish either of the two, not only will you be infusing the right amount of effort and make the food come to its full potential, but you will be saving more time and money as well.

The Slow Crock-Pot

a. It consists of three parts: the lid, the round oval pot, and heater on the sides and bottom.

b. It uses moisture instead of heat to cook the food for a long period of time.

c. It takes its time cooking — it doesn't have any other temperature setting other than HIGH/LOW.

d. It helps kill bacteria due to its tightly covered lid. It works best for cooking processed food.

e. It is best used when using hard types of meat.

The Slow Cooker

a. Its heating element is found at the bottom — there are none on the sides.

b. It has more temperature settings.

c. It works best with stews, soups, and everything else that is much smaller in cuts.

d. The heating inside it is not continuous. It runs in cycles, turning on and off for certain periods of time

In the process of slow cooking, you will need to know what's best for the type of food you'll be making — you need to distinguish whether the dish will cook better in a Crock-Pot or slow cooker.

Slow cooking is good for dishes that require an even level of it being cooked. It requires a bit of carefulness in order for your dish to achieve good quality so you have to bear in mind the type of pot you'll be using.

Here are also some strategies you can keep in mind when using these equipment to help save on time and effort and maximize the benefits of the slow cooking method.

o Avoid a dish that requires a lot of pre-preparation. More often than not, these are the types of dishes that will require more ingredients to be added later on.

o Prepare everything you need the night before. Doing this works best if you're on the go. Plus, it's a good way to ensure that you don't forget stuff.

o It's best to use inexpensive types of meat. Slow cooking makes everything tender. You won't notice the difference, and you get to save money.

o Do not add too much liquid. Two-third full is usually the ideal amount.

o For soups, you can stir in a small amount of flour to thicken.

o It is best to always use the LOW setting.

o Always cut the meat or vegetables in the right size so the heat can evenly cook them.

o Resist the urge to peek from time to time as removing the lid causes heat to escape, thus prolonging your cooking time.

o Make sure that the Crock-Pot or slow cooker that you are using is of top quality to avoid any inconvenience.

Chapter 3: Three-Vegetable Combinations

A vegetable slow cooked recipe almost never fails to impress. Whether you're trying to better your health or simply just enjoying the goodness of slowly cooked flavor-rich veggies, slow cooked vegetable recipes are always on top of every recipe list.

A three-vegetable ingredient combination is not bad for starters. It's convenient and delicious at the same time. This brings out the advantage of slow cooking because vegetables in any combination are nice and nutritious.

And despite what most people think, slow cooking does not take out the nutrients in vegetables as long as they are prepared correctly. If done right, slow cooking has a very minimal effect on the nutrient levels of the vegetables you are preparing.

There are groups of vegetables that actually retain more of their health benefits and disease-fighting components when exposed to slow heat. This is actually beneficial to moms who have to cater to picky eaters. Slow cooking makes vegetables more appealing and at the same time, nutritious.

The Right Kind Of Vegetables

There are some vegetables that are actually best infused with slow cooking. Vegetables like carrots, tomatoes, broccoli, cabbage, and kale are the best examples of those leaves that retain their antioxidant qualities when exposed to slow heat.

Slow cooking is a very gentle method of cooking vegetables compared to any other method. All you need to do to prepare everything correctly is to make sure that the pot temperature is always at its lowest to induce rich flavors and evenly cook the veggies without sacrificing the health benefit they bring.

Here are a few starter recipes you might enjoy with the best three-vegetable combination:

Potatoes, Carrots, Cabbage Soup

You will need:

1 large potato, peeled and cut in cubes

1 whole carrot, peeled and diced in cubes

1/2 slice whole cabbage, cut into strips

1 onion, cut in half

Other ingredients:

4 cups beef broth

2 cups milk/cream

Preparation:

Stir in the beef broth in the pot together with the vegetables. Cook slowly until potatoes are tender. Add milk/cream and let simmer again for 5 to 10 minutes. Put in a bowl and serve.

Sweet Potatoes, Bell Pepper, Zucchini Roast

You will need:

2 bell peppers

1 large sweet potato, peeled and cut in cubes

3 zucchini sticks

Other ingredients:

5 cloves garlic, peeled

Salt/herb to taste

Preparation:

Grease the pot and add in the vegetables. Season evenly as desired. Cook in low temperature for 3 to 4 hours. It is served best with brown rice or grilled meat.

Broccoli, Cauliflower, Green Beans

You will need:

1 cup fresh broccoli stems

1 cup cauliflower stems

1 cup green beans

Other ingredients:

Salt to taste

Butter for flavor

1/2 cup water

Preparation:

Grease pot with butter and add in vegetables. Season with salt. Add water and cook in low temperature for 4 to 5 hours. Serve.

There are other vegetables that you can combine to make a unique three-ingredient Crock-Pot recipe. Improvising while keeping everything simple will make slow cooking more convenient and enjoyable.

Chapter 4: Slow Cooking Meat

Cooking meat in a slow cooker is really as easy as it looks. Slow cookers are very much economical and practical when it comes to preparing meat dishes for the whole family to enjoy.

Preparing this with a slow cooker or Crock-Pot will save you money due to the fact that slow cookers can turn any tough meat into a fabulous tender roast while you wait in the comfort of your home.

Here's the secret: "Tough" meats are usually more budget-friendly because they have more ligaments in the meat than the other meat parts.

Those tough parts are tenderized during the slow cooking process so you really won't have any problem in that department if you're using a slow cooker.

The slower the cooking, the better the results are. Slow cooking tenderizes and breaks down that protein ligament which increases the savory taste.

Here are a few tips and strategies that you can use to make slow cooking even better:

1. Save effort and time in the long run by browning the meat first before putting it together to balance out the taste.

2. Marinade or prepare the meat and condiments that will be used the night before to simmer in the flavor inside the meat before cooking.

3. Save more money by using these parts instead: beef brisket, chicken thighs, pork and lamb shoulders, etc.

4. Remove the fat before cooking. The fats in meat do not melt away unless fried.

5. Avoid putting too much water. About 3/4 is enough. Do this to make the broth more concentrated. This provides a richer taste.

Here are a few samples of three-ingredient meat slow cooking recipes to give you more cooking ideas in the long run:

Beef Tacos

You will need:

1 pound beef

1 sachet taco seasoning

1 10-ounce can tomatoes

Preparation:

It's super easy! Put everything in the slow cooker and mix well to induce an even flavor. Cook in low temperature for 5 to 6 hours. Serve with taco shells.

Chicken Salsa

You will need:

Chicken fillet

1 can condensed cheddar soup

1 jar salsa

Preparation:

Put everything in the slow cooker and let cook for 8 to 9 hours over low temperature. Serve.

Garlic Buttered Fish

You will need:

4 strips fish fillet of your choice

2 tablespoons butter

2 tablespoons garlic cloves, minced

Salt and pepper to taste

Preparation:

Pull out a large sheet of aluminum foil and place the fish fillets on top. Add salt and pepper. Add butter and garlic cloves evenly against the fish. Wrap and put inside the slow cooker. Cook for about 4 to 5 hours over low heat. Serve.

When it comes to slow cooking meat, the sky is pretty much the limit. There are several easy recipes you can try and improvise some of the ingredients that are needed to give your dish its unique signature taste. You can actually have more fun trying more stuff than sticking to basic recipes. Go crazy and explore more options!

Chapter 5: Everyday Three-Ingredient Recipes

The best thing to keep in mind if you're planning to make an everyday three-ingredient recipe for the family is to always choose the best possible ingredients you can buy or find in the market.

One great strategy that you can use to lessen the preparation time is to use enhanced products or double-made products as an ingredient, as they work best to save on money as well.

Enhanced products such as mixed vegetables, marinated meat, garlic butter, tomatoes with chili, garlic chili, and many more are perfect for slow cooking. You can always find one to mix and match with your recipe in your local grocery or market.

Any kind of vegetable and meat combination will more than likely work if cooked with a slow cooker. You'll have all the variations you can choose from, depending on your mood. Fresh vegetables or frozen vegetables are okay to use.

However, dishes with minimal ingredients need help when it comes to extra flavoring. Adding a dab of butter or seasoning to any of your desired recipe will really work wonders for the dish.

For meat dishes, a dab of soy sauce always works well. A teaspoon of oyster or Worcestershire sauce while simmering gives a good Oriental twist to the dish you're making. The options of what you can do or add are actually endless as long as you know what type of dish you want to serve.

Dairy products also work well with slow cookers. Soups are always good with cream and eggs make for good Oriental soups. Cheese and vegetables are also a good combination for slow cooking. Melted cheese will make any dish extra delicious.

Here are some good yet simple recipes for you to try:

Beef, String Beans, Tomatoes

You will need:

Beef strips or beef brisket

A handful string beans

2 tomatoes, diced in half

Other ingredients:

4 tablespoons soy sauce

2 tablespoons oyster sauce

Pepper to taste

Preparation:

Put the beef brisket/strips with the tomatoes and stir in the sauces. Cook for 8 hours. Add string beans and simmer for 10 more minutes for a crunchy, veggie twist. Serve and enjoy!

Chicken, Cheese, Peas

You will need:

Chicken fillet

Cheese (the right amount suited for your taste), cut in cubes

A handful frozen peas

Other ingredients:

1 teaspoon butter

Salt and pepper to taste

Preparation:

Brown chicken meat first in a skillet and then place in the slow cooker. Add in vegetables and cheese cubes, making sure to spread evenly. Add salt and pepper to taste. Add the butter and cook for 5 to 6 hours. Serve.

Onions, Eggs, Celery

You will need:

1 whole white onion, diced

2 whole eggs

Celery sticks, diced

Other ingredients:

Salt and pepper to taste

Flour cornstarch to thicken sauce

Beef or chicken broth

Preparation:

Stir in beef or chicken broth into the pot. Add in eggs and stir accordingly. Add onions and celery. Put in 1 teaspoon of cornstarch or flour to thicken. Stir to even out surface. Cook for 4 to 5 hours. Serves.

Chicken Thighs, Potatoes, Garlic

You will need:

Chicken drumsticks

1 whole potato, cut into cubes

3 cloves garlic, peeled and minced

Other ingredients:

½ cup soy sauce

½ cup vinegar

Salt and sugar

Preparation:

Put chicken, garlic, and potatoes in the slow cooker and add in the sauce, sugar, and salt to taste. Cook for 5 to 6 hours. Serve.

These are just a few varieties of the endless things you can do and combine with a slow cooker. You can try to improvise and create your own version of soups and dishes. Once you get the hang of it, you can slowly transition to more ingredients and experiment with different dishes.

Chapter 6: Safety Precautions For Slow Cooking

With all of the wonderful things you've learned so far on how to make slow cooking simple and easy, and how you can create convenient and delicious meals with just three ingredients, you must also be mindful there are always pros and cons while doing so.

Just because a certain equipment or tool is convenient and easy to use doesn't mean you can be careless with it. Great cooking also considers safety precautions to avoid any inconveniences, injuries, and accidents in the kitchen.

Using the slow cooker is no different than using any typical kitchen equipment. You always have to be careful while using it so it won't, by any chance, become hazardous to you and your family's health and well-being.

Every safety measure in the kitchen always starts with a clean space for you to place the cooker on. Since bacteria thrive everywhere, there is a chance that the food might get contaminated right after cooking and exposure to air. Make sure the area is sanitized to avoid getting any unnecessary "ingredient" added to the dish.

Also, the heat of the cooker must always be at a certain bacteria-killing temperature. Therefore, when cooking on low temperature, you have to make sure that the food reaches an evenly cooked state.

And to make sure that the food reaches top quality, preparing the meat separately from the vegetables is a must. Do not put frozen meat into the pot as it risks the meat not being cooked 100% all the way.

Another thing that you might consider is to not put overly large chunks of meat or vegetable cuts more than your slow cooker can handle. The safest is 2/3 full of the pot to ensure everything cooks through. It is good to cut the meat in a much smaller portion since large chunks of meat take longer to cook.

Take note to always keep the lid closed while cooking. The heat trapped inside is important in making everything go well together so try and avoid peeping unless you really need to check on your dish.

Lastly, choose dishes that have a higher level of moisture as an everyday recipe for the pot such as soups, stews, and the like. The steam from the moisture helps kill any present bacteria, giving your dish just the right amount of awesomeness and healthiness before serving.

Conclusion

Thank you again for downloading this book!

Slow cooking works wonders in preparing meals without much hassle or effort on your part. There are other several ways on how you can get the most out of it and various ways on how you can improve the sample recipes provided.

Once you've gotten comfortable with the basics, then you can create and combine your own unique ingredients to make the perfect dish! Dare to be creative enough to experiment on certain ingredients and explore different flavors. Just remember to handle everything with care and have fun along the way.

Part -2

INTRODUCTION

SLOW COOKER *IS NOT SLOW!*

low cooker recipes are great for people who like creative and modern food, similar to what would be served in a good restaurant.

Meals can be assembled early in the morning and consumed shortly upon arrival home. It's even faster than getting takeout!

What is a Slow Cooker? A Slow Cooker also known as a Crock-Pot is a counter top electrical cooking appliance that is used for simmering, which requires maintaining a relatively low temperature, allowing unattended cooking for many hours.

Slow cookers can be used to make main dishes, one-pot meals, side dishes, even desserts. In most cases recipes need only a few minutes of prep time and zero intervention time during the cooking.

Look for slow cookers that have at least a low and high setting. This is standard for the medium/large-size models, but many 2-quart models only have an on/off option.

Appetizers and Snacks

CRANBERRY TURKEY MEATBALLS

APPETIZERS AND SNACKS › TURKEY MEATBALLS, CHILI SAUCE, CRANBERRY SAUCE, BROWN SUGAR

SERVES: 12

28 ounces frozen, precooked turkey meatballs (about 24 meatballs)

1/4 cup chili sauce

3 cups whole-berry Cranberry Sauce

1 1/2 tablespoons dark brown sugar

1 tablespoon ginger preserves

Defrost the meatballs according to package instructions. Mix together the chili sauce, cranberry sauce, sugar, and preserves in a large bowl.

Pour half of the sauce into the bottom of a 4-quart oval slow cooker. Place the meatballs on top. Pour the remaining sauce over the meatballs. Cook on low for 4 hours or on high for 2.

CHICKEN BITES

APPETIZERS AND SNACKS › CHICKEN BREASTS, ONION, GARLIC, CHILI, RASPBERRY JAM, WORCESTERSHIRE SAUCE, BALSAMIC VINEGAR

SERVES: 16

2 pounds boneless skinless chicken breasts, cubed

1 onion, minced

2 cloves garlic, minced

1/2 cup chili sauce

1/2 cup no-sugar raspberry jam

1 tablespoon Worcestershire sauce

1 tablespoon balsamic vinegar

Place the chicken into a 4-quart slow cooker. In a small bowl, whisk together the onion, garlic, chili sauce, jam, Worcestershire sauce, and balsamic vinegar. Pour it over the meat.

Cook on low for 3 hours or until the chicken is cooked through. Stir before serving.

CURRIED CHICKEN BREASTS

APPETIZERS AND SNACKS › ONION, GARLIC, GINGER, CURRY, CHICKEN BROTH, TAPIOCA, CHICKEN BREASTS, YOGURT, CILANTRO, ALMONDS

SERVES: 6

2 onions, minced

6 garlic cloves, minced

2 tablespoons minced or grated fresh ginger

4 teaspoons curry powder

1 tablespoon vegetable oil

1 tablespoon tomato paste

1 cup low-sodium chicken broth

3 tablespoons Minute tapioca

6 (12-ounce) bone-in split chicken breasts, skin removed, trimmed

sea salt and freshly ground black pepper

1/2 cup raisins

1/2 cup plain whole-milk yogurt

2 tablespoons minced fresh cilantro

1/2 cup sliced almonds, toasted

Microwave onions, garlic, ginger, curry powder, oil, and tomato paste in bowl, stirring occasionally, until onions are softened, about 5 minutes; transfer to slow cooker.

Stir broth and tapioca into slow cooker. Season chicken with salt and pepper and nestle into slow cooker. Cover and cook until chicken is tender, 4 to 6 hours on low.

Gently stir in raisins and let sit until heated through, about 10 minutes. Transfer chicken to serving platter and tent loosely with aluminum foil. Let braising liquid settle for 5 minutes, then remove fat from surface using large spoon.

In bowl, combine 1/4 cup hot braising liquid with yogurt (to temper), then stir mixture back into slow cooker. Stir in cilantro and season with salt and pepper to taste. Spoon 1 cup sauce over chicken, sprinkle with almonds, and serve with remaining sauce.

BALSAMIC ALMONDS

APPETIZERS AND SNACKS › ALMONDS, BROWN SUGAR, BALSAMIC VINEGAR, KOSHER SALT

SERVES: 15

2 cups whole almonds

1/2 cup dark brown sugar

1/2 cup balsamic vinegar

1/2 teaspoon kosher salt

Place all ingredients into a 4-quart oval slow cooker. Cook uncovered on high for 4 hours, stirring every 15 minutes or until all the liquid has evaporated. The almonds will have a syrupy coating.

Line two cookie sheets with parchment paper. Pour the almonds in a single layer on the baking sheets to cool completely. Store in an airtight container for up to 1 week.

STICKY WINGS

APPETIZERS AND SNACKS › BROWN SUGAR, SOY SAUCE, GINGER, GARLIC, CAYENNE, CHICKEN WINGS, TOMATO PASTE

SERVES: 4-6

3/4 cup packed dark brown sugar

1/4 cup soy sauce

2 tablespoons minced or grated fresh ginger

4 garlic cloves, minced

1/2 teaspoon cayenne pepper

4 pounds whole chicken wings, wingtips discarded and wings split

sea salt and freshly ground black pepper

vegetable oil spray

1/4 cup water

1/4 cup tomato paste

Stir 1/4 cup sugar, 1 tablespoon soy sauce, ginger, garlic, and 1/4 teaspoon cayenne into slow cooker. Season chicken with salt and pepper, add to slow cooker, and toss to coat. Cover and cook until chicken is tender, about 4 hours on low.

Position oven rack 10 inches from broiler element and heat broiler. Place wire rack in aluminum foil–lined rimmed baking sheet and coat with vegetable oil spray. Transfer chicken to prepared baking sheet; discard braising liquid.

Combine remaining 1/2 cup sugar, water, tomato paste, remaining 3 tablespoons soy sauce, and remaining 1/4 teaspoon cayenne in bowl. Brush chicken with half of mixture and broil until lightly charred and crisp, 10 to 15 minutes. Flip chicken over, brush with remaining mixture, and continue to broil until lightly charred and crisp on second side, 5 to 10 minutes longer. Serve.

BUFFALO MEATBALLS

SERVES: 8

1 pound ground organic chicken

2 ounces cream cheese, softened

2 large eggs

2 tablespoons celery, chopped fine

1 to 3 tablespoons crumbled blue cheese (to taste)

1/2 teaspoon black pepper

SAUCE:

1/2 cup coconut oil or butter

1/2 cup hot sauce

RANCH DRESSING:

8 ounces cream cheese

1/2 cup organic chicken or beef broth

1/2 teaspoon dried chives

1/2 teaspoon dried parsley

1/2 teaspoon dried dill weed

1/4 teaspoon garlic powder

1/4 teaspoon onion powder

1/8 teaspoon Celtic sea salt

1/8 teaspoon ground black pepper

In a medium bowl combine the ground chicken, cream cheese, eggs, celery, blue cheese and pepper. The mixture will be sticky. Form 1 inch balls.

Place in a 4-quart slow cooker on medium for 2-3 hours.

Once the meatballs are done, add in the butter and hot sauce, stir to coat the meatballs.

Leave in slow cooker on very low for your guests to enjoy. Serve with the Ranch dressing and celery sticks.

MEXICAN MEATBALLS

APPETIZERS AND SNACKS › BEEF, CHICKEN, CUMIN, CILANTRO, GARLIC, ONION, EGG, SALSA

SERVES: 8

1 pound grass fed ground beef

1/2 pound organic ground chicken

1 1/4 teaspoon cumin seasoning

1 tablespoon coconut flour

1/4 cup chopped fresh cilantro

2 cloves garlic, minced

1/2 cup onion, chopped

1 egg, beaten

1 (28-ounces) jar salsa

In a bowl, mix the ground beef, ground chicken, cumin, coconut flour, cilantro, garlic, onion, and egg. Shape the mixture into 16 meatballs.

Place the meatballs in a 4-quart slow cooker. Cook on Low for 6 to 8 hours. Drain any fat from the slow cooker.

Place the salsa in the slow cooker over the meatballs. Serve with guacamole.

SNACK MIX

SERVES: 8

2 tablespoons melted butter

1 teaspoon garlic powder

1 teaspoon onion powder

1 teaspoon paprika

1 teaspoon dried thyme

1 teaspoon dill weed

1 teaspoon chili powder

1 teaspoon Worcestershire sauce

1 1/2 cups crispy corn cereal squares

1 1/2 cups crispy wheat cereal squares

1 1/2 cups crispy rice cereal squares

1 cup pretzel wheels

1 cup roasted peanuts or almonds

Pour the butter, spices, and Worcestershire sauce into the bottom of a 6-quart slow cooker. Stir. Add the cereal, pretzels, and nuts. Cook uncovered on low for 2–3 hours, stirring every 30 minutes.

Pour onto a baking sheet and allow to cool. Store in an airtight container.

Soups and Stews

VEGGIE BEEF SOUP

SOUPS AND STEWS › BEEF, CARROTS, POTATOES, ONION, TOMATOES, PEAS, THYME

SERVES: 4

1 pound boneless beef chuck roast, cubed or lean ground beef

2 cups carrots, sliced

2 medium potatoes, peeled and largely diced

1 medium onion, chopped

2 (14 ounces) cans diced tomatoes with juice

1 cup water

8 ounces frozen peas

1/2 teaspoon sea salt

1/2 teaspoon dried thyme

In a large slow cooker, combine beef, carrots, potatoes, onions, tomatoes with juice, salt, thyme, and water. Stir well.

Cover and cook on low heat for 8 hours. About 30 minutes before serving, stir in peas and allow to soften. Serve warm.

THAI CHICKEN SOUP

SOUPS AND STEWS › CHICKEN THIGHS, ONION, GARLIC, GINGER, CHICKEN BROTH, CARROTS, CILANTRO, MUSHROOMS, THAI REC CURRY

SERVES: 6-8

2 onions, minced

6 garlic cloves, minced

2 tablespoons minced or grated fresh ginger

1 tablespoon vegetable oil

4 cups low-sodium chicken broth

2 (14-ounce) cans coconut milk

2 stalks lemon grass, bottom 5 inches only, bruised

2 carrots, peeled and sliced 1/4 inch thick

3 tablespoons fish sauce

10 cilantro stems, tied together with twine

1 1/2 pounds boneless, skinless chicken thighs, trimmed

sea salt and freshly ground black pepper

8 ounces white mushrooms, trimmed and sliced thin

3 tablespoons fresh lime juice from 2 limes

1 tablespoon sugar

2 teaspoons Thai red curry paste

GARNISHES

1/2 cup fresh cilantro leaves

2 fresh Thai, serrano, or jalapeño chiles, stemmed, seeded and sliced thin

2 scallions, sliced thin

Lime wedges, for serving

Microwave onions, garlic, ginger, and oil in bowl, stirring occasionally, until onions are softened, about 5 minutes; transfer to slow cooker.

Stir broth, 1 can coconut milk, lemon grass, carrots, 1 tablespoon fish sauce, and cilantro stems into slow cooker. Season chicken with salt and pepper and nestle into slow cooker. Cover and cook until chicken is tender, 4 to 6 hours on low.

Transfer chicken to cutting board, let cool slightly, then shred into bite-size pieces. Let soup settle for 5 minutes, then remove fat from surface using large spoon. Discard lemon grass and cilantro stems.

Stir in mushrooms, cover, and cook on high until mushrooms are tender, 5 to 15 minutes. Microwave remaining can coconut milk in bowl until hot, about 3 minutes, then whisk in remaining 2 tablespoons fish sauce, lime juice, sugar, and curry paste to dissolve.

Stir hot coconut milk mixture and shredded chicken into soup and let sit until heated through, about 5 minutes. Season with salt and pepper to taste and serve with garnishes.

SPLIT PEA SOUP

SOUPS AND STEWS › SPLIT PEAS, CARROT, PARSNIP, CELERY, ONION, SHALLOT, HAM STEAK, SAGE, DILL WEED, CELERY SEED, CAYENNE

SERVES: 6

1/2 cup green split peas

1/2 cup yellow split peas

1 large carrot, diced

1 large parsnip, diced

1 stalk celery, diced

1 medium onion, diced

2 shallots, minced

4 ounces 98% fat-free ham steak, diced

1 teaspoon minced fresh sage

1/4 teaspoon dill weed

1/4 teaspoon celery seed

1/4 teaspoon ground cayenne

1 teaspoon hickory liquid smoke

1/2 teaspoon celery flakes

1/2 teaspoon dried chervil

5 cups water

Place all ingredients into a 4-quart slow cooker. Stir. Cook on low for 12–15 hours.

If the soup is wetter than desired, uncover and cook on high for 30 minutes before serving.

CREAM OF MUSHROOM SOUP

SOUPS AND STEWS › MUSHROOMS, LEMON JUICE, SHALLOTS, THYME, BAY LEAF, CREAM CHEESE

SERVES: 4

1 pound button mushrooms, cleaned and sliced

1 tablespoon lemon juice

2 tablespoons minced shallots

1 teaspoon dried thyme

1/2 bay leaf

1 teaspoon sea salt

1/2 teaspoon freshly ground black pepper

4 ounces cream cheese

2 cups veggie or chicken broth

In a food processor, coarsely chop mushrooms in lemon juice. Add all the ingredients to a slow cooker on medium for 4 to 8 hours. You may need to whisk in the cream cheese in to incorporate it well. Add salt and pepper to taste.

CURRIED EGGPLANT SOUP

SOUPS AND STEWS › EGGPLANT, DICED TOMATOES, ONION, GRANNY SMITH APPLE, CURRY, SOY SAUCE, HONEY, VEGETABLE BROTH

SERVES: 4

1 large (2-pound) eggplant, peeled and diced

1 (14.5-ounce) can diced tomatoes, undrained

1 onion, diced

1 Granny Smith or other tart green apple, peeled and diced

2 tablespoons curry powder

1 tablespoon soy sauce

1 tablespoon honey

1/4 teaspoon kosher salt

1/4 teaspoon cayenne pepper

4 cups vegetable broth

FOR TOPPING:

feta cheese, chopped fresh cilantro leaves

Use a 4-quart slow cooker. Add the eggplant, tomatoes, onion, and apple to the insert. Add the curry powder, soy sauce, honey, salt, and cayenne pepper.

Stir in the broth. Cover, and cook on low for 7 to 8 hours. Before serving, blend with a handheld immersion blender until you have reached desired consistency or let cool a bit and blend in small batches in a traditional blender.

Add cheese and cilantro to each bowl, if desired.

LENTIL AND LAMB SOUP

SOUPS AND STEWS › LAMB SHOULDER, ONION, GARLIC, RED PEPPER, BROWN LENTILS, CHICKEN BROTH, PARSLEY

SERVES: 6-8

2 tablespoons extra-virgin olive oil

2 pounds lamb shoulder, excess fat trimmed, and cut into 1-in pieces

sea salt

1 large onion, finely chopped

2 garlic cloves, minced

1/2 teaspoons red pepper flakes

2 cups brown lentils, rinsed and picked over for stones

one 14 1/2- to 15-ounces can chopped tomatoes, with their juice

8 cups chicken broth

1/2 cup chopped fresh flat-leaf parsley

freshly ground black pepper (optional)

In a large skillet, heat the olive oil over medium-high heat. Sprinkle the lamb with 1 1/2 teaspoons salt. Brown the lamb, a few pieces at a time, transferring the browned meat to the insert of a 5- to 7-quart slow cooker.

When all the lamb has been browned, add the onion, garlic, and red pepper flakes to the skillet, and cook for 3 minutes, until the onion begins to soften.

Transfer the mixture to the slow cooker, and stir in the lentils, tomatoes, and broth.

Cover and cook on high for 3 hours, or on low for 6 hours. The lamb will be tender.

Skim any excess fat from the surface of the soup and add the parsley. Taste for seasoning and add more salt and some black pepper, if you like, before serving.

VEGGIE CHILI

SOUPS AND STEWS › CARROTS, CELERY, ONION, MUSHROOMS, ZUCCHINI,

SQUASH, CHILI, PEPPER, BASIL, TOMATO, BEANS

SERVES: 15

1 cup carrots, chopped

1 cup celery, chopped

1 medium onion, chopped

16 ounces sliced fresh mushrooms, sliced

1 large zucchini, chopped

1 yellow squash, chopped

1 tablespoon chili powder

1 teaspoon seasoned pepper

1 teaspoon dried basil

24 ounces tomato juice

8 ounces can tomato sauce

2 (14-ounces) cans diced tomatoes, undrained

1 (15-ounces) can pinto beans, rinsed and drained

1 (15-ounces) can northern beans, rinsed and drained

1 (15-ounces) can black beans, rinsed and drained

1 (15-ounces) can red kidney beans, rinsed and drained

8 ounces frozen corn

Place all Ingredients into a large slow cooker and stir until well mixed. Cover and cook on low for 6 to 8 hours or until veggies are tender and the soup is thickened. Serve warm.

TEX-MEX CHICKEN STEW

SOUPS AND STEWS › ONION, JALAPENO, GARLIC, TOMATO PASTE, CHILI, TAPIOCA, CHICKEN THIGHS, CORN, BLACK BEANS, CILANTRO

SERVES: 6-8

2 onions, minced

2 jalapeño chiles, stemmed, seeded, and minced

6 garlic cloves, minced

1 tablespoon tomato paste

1 tablespoon vegetable oil

1 tablespoon chili powder

4 cups low-sodium chicken broth, plus extra as needed

1 (14.5-ounce) can diced tomatoes, drained

1/4 cup Minute tapioca

1 tablespoon light brown sugar

3 pounds boneless, skinless chicken thighs, trimmed

sea salt and freshly ground black pepper

2 cups frozen corn

1 (15-ounce) can black beans, drained and rinsed

minced canned chipotle chile in adobo sauce

1/4 cup minced fresh cilantro

Microwave onions, jalapeños, garlic, tomato paste, oil, and chili powder in bowl, stirring occasionally, until onions are softened, about 5 minutes; transfer to slow cooker.

Stir broth, tomatoes, tapioca, and sugar into slow cooker. Season chicken with salt and pepper and nestle into slow cooker. Cover and cook until chicken is tender, 4 to 6 hours on low.

Transfer chicken to cutting board, let cool slightly, then shred into bite-size pieces. Let stew settle for 5 minutes, then remove fat from surface using large spoon.

Stir in corn and beans, cover, and cook on high until heated through, about 10 minutes. Stir in shredded chicken, chipotles to taste, and let sit until heated through, about 5 minutes. (Adjust stew consistency with additional hot broth as needed.) Stir in cilantro, season with salt and pepper to taste, and serve.

ROSEMARY-THYME STEW

SOUPS AND STEWS › ONION, CARROT, CELERY, GARLIC, POTATOES, THYME, ROSEMARY, CHICKEN BREASTS

SERVES: 4

1 teaspoon canola oil

1 large onion, diced

1 tablespoon flour

1 carrot, diced

2 stalks celery, diced

2 cloves garlic, minced

1 cup diced Yukon Gold potatoes

3 1/2 tablespoons minced fresh thyme

3 tablespoons minced fresh rosemary

1 pound boneless skinless chicken breast, cut into 1 inch cubes

1/4 teaspoon salt

1/2 teaspoon freshly ground black pepper

1 1/2 cup water or Chicken Stock

1/2 cup frozen or fresh corn kernels

Heat the oil in a large skillet. Sauté the onion, flour, carrots, celery, garlic, potatoes, thyme, rosemary, and chicken until the chicken is white on all sides. Drain off any excess fat.

Put sautéed ingredients into a 4-quart slow cooker. Sprinkle with salt and pepper. Pour in the water or stock. Stir. Cook for 8–9 hours on low.

Add the corn. Cover and cook an additional 1/2 hour on high. Stir before serving.

SPICY BEEF STEW

SOUPS AND STEWS › BEEF, GARLIC, GINGER, JALAPENO, CURRY, ONION

SERVES: 4

1 tablespoon coconut oil

1 pound grass fed beef stew meat

sea salt and pepper to taste

2 cloves garlic, minced

1 teaspoons chopped fresh ginger

1 fresh jalapeño peppers, diced

1 tablespoon curry powder

1 (14.5-ounces) can diced tomatoes with juice

1 onion, sliced and quartered

1 cup organic beef broth

Heat the oil in a skillet over medium heat, and brown the beef on all sides. Remove from skillet, reserving juices, and season with salt and pepper.

Cook and stir the garlic, ginger, and jalapeño in the skillet for 2 minutes, until tender, and season with curry powder. Mix in the diced tomatoes and juice.

Place the onion in the bottom of a slow cooker, and layer with the browned beef. Scoop the skillet mixture in the slow cooker, and mix in the beef broth.

Cover, and cook 6 to 8 hours on low.

GREEK STEW

SOUPS AND STEWS › CHICKEN THIGHS, CAULIFLOWER, RED ONION, GARLIC,

CHICKEN BROTH, CINNAMON, THYME, KALAMATA OLIVES

SERVES: 6

2 pounds boneless, skinless chicken thighs (frozen is fine)

1 small head cauliflower, stem removed and florets separated

1 red onion, diced

6 garlic cloves, minced

1 (28-ounce) can diced tomatoes, undrained

1 cup chicken broth

1 tablespoon red wine vinegar

1/2 teaspoon ground cinnamon

1/2 teaspoon dried thyme

1/4 teaspoon ground black pepper

1/3 cup pitted Kalamata olives

1/4 cup crumbled feta cheese (optional)

Use a 6-quart slow cooker. Place the chicken into the insert. Add the cauliflower, onion, and garlic. Pour in the tomatoes and broth. Stir in the vinegar, cinnamon, thyme, and pepper. Drop in the olives, and cover. Cook on low for 8 hours, or until the chicken breaks apart easily with a fork. Serve in large bowls with the cheese, if desired.

Meats

ITALIAN CHICKEN

MEATS › CHICKEN BREAST, MUSHROOMS, ITALIAN DRESSING, WHITE WINE, CREAM CHEESE, BUTTER, PAPRIKA

SERVES: 6

6 boneless skinless chicken breasts

16 ounces Baby Portabella mushrooms, sliced

1 packet dry Italian dressing mix

1 cup white wine

1 8-ounces package fat free cream cheese (room temperature)

8 ounces fat free chicken broth

1 tablespoon butter

2 teaspoons paprika

In a medium sauce pan, melt butter then whisk in wine, chicken broth, dressing mix, and cream cheese until smooth. Place mushrooms and chicken in the bottom of a large slow cooker. Pour wine sauce over the chicken. Cover and cook on low for 6 hours.

AMERICAN POT ROAST

MEATS › GARLIC POWDER, BASIL, POT ROAST, POTATO, ONION, CELERY, CARROT

SERVES: 6

1 tablespoon garlic powder

2 teaspoons dried basil

1 teaspoon kosher salt

1/2 teaspoon freshly ground black pepper

1 (4-pound) pot roast, trimmed

6 red potatoes, washed and quartered

2 onions, cut into wedges

1 bunch celery, cut into 1-inch pieces

1 cup carrots cut into 1-inch pieces

2 cups beef broth

Use a 6-quart slow cooker. In a small bowl, combine the garlic powder, basil, salt, and pepper. Rub the spices into the meat, taking care to cover all sides. Place the meat into the insert. Nestle all the vegetables around the meat. Pour in the broth. Cover, and cook on low for 8 to 10 hours, or until the meat has relaxed and pulls apart easily with a fork.

PEPPER VENISON STEAK

MEATS › VENISON SIRLOIN, GARLIC, BEEF BROTH, ONION, BELL PEPPER

SERVES: 8

2 pounds venison sirloin, cut in 2-inch strips

2 cloves garlic, roasted and smashed

3 tablespoons coconut oil

1/2 cup organic beef broth

1/2 teaspoon guar gum (thickener)

1/2 cup chopped onion

1 red bell pepper, sliced

1 green bell peppers, sliced

1 (14.5-ounces) jar stewed tomatoes, with liquid

3 tablespoons coconut aminos

1 tablespoon Swerve, Granular (or equivalent)

1 teaspoon sea salt

Use a 6-quart slow cooker. In a small bowl, combine the garlic powder, basil, salt, and pepper. Rub the spices into the meat, taking care to cover all sides. Place the meat into the insert. Nestle all the vegetables around the meat. Pour in the broth. Cover, and cook on low for 8 to 10 hours, or until the meat has relaxed and pulls apart easily with a fork.

ROULADE

MEATS › RED WINE, STEAKS, MUSTARD, BACON CRUMBLES

SERVES: 4

1/4 cup red wine

1 cup water

4 very thin round steaks (about 3/4 pound total)

2 tablespoons grainy German-style mustard

1 tablespoon lean bacon crumbles (optional)

4 dill pickle spears

Pour the wine and water into the bottom of an oval 4-quart slow cooker.

Place the steaks horizontally on a platter. Spread 1/2 tablespoon mustard on each steak and sprinkle with one-quarter of the bacon crumbles. Place one of the pickle spears on one end of each steak. Roll each steak toward the other end, so it looks like a spiral. Place on a skillet seam-side down. Cook for 1 minute, then use tongs to flip the steaks carefully and cook the other side for 1 minute.

Place each roll in a single layer in the water-wine mixture. Cook on low for 1 hour. Remove the rolls, discarding the cooking liquid.

EASY BARBECUED RIBS

MEATS › PAPRIKA, CAYENNE, BROWN SUGAR, PORK BABY BACK RIBS, BARBECUE SAUCE

SERVES: 6-8

3 tablespoons sweet paprika

2 tablespoons brown sugar

1/4 teaspoon cayenne pepper

sea salt and freshly ground black pepper

6 pounds pork baby back ribs

3 cups barbecue sauce

vegetable oil spray

Mix paprika, sugar, cayenne, 1 tablespoon salt, and 1 tablespoon pepper together, then rub mixture evenly over ribs. Arrange ribs upright in slow cooker, with meaty sides facing outward (see photo). Pour barbecue sauce over ribs, cover, and cook until ribs are tender, 6 to 8 hours on low.

Position oven rack 10 inches from broiler element and heat broiler. Place wire rack in aluminum foil–lined rimmed baking sheet and coat with vegetable oil spray. Carefully transfer ribs, meaty side down, to prepared baking sheet and tent with foil. Let braising liquid settle for 5 minutes, then remove fat from surface using large spoon.

Strain braising liquid into medium saucepan and simmer until thickened and measures 2 cups, 15 to 20 minutes. Season with salt and pepper to taste.

Brush ribs with some sauce and broil until beginning to brown, 2 to 4 minutes. Flip ribs over, brush with more sauce, and continue to broil until ribs are well browned and sticky, 9 to 12 minutes longer, brushing with additional sauce every few minutes.

Transfer ribs to cutting board, tent with foil, and let rest for 10 minutes. Serve with remaining sauce.

MEAT LOAF

MEATS › GROUND BEEF, TURKEY BREAST, MUSHROOMS, ITALIAN SEASONING, ONION, KETCHUP, DIJON MUSTARD

SERVES: 8

1 cup of whole wheat bread crumbs

1 pound lean ground beef

1 pound ground turkey breast

1 teaspoon dried Italian seasoning

1 cup fresh button mushrooms, sliced

1 small onion, diced

3/4 teaspoon sea salt

2 large eggs, beaten

2 garlic cloves, minced

3 tablespoons ketchup

2 teaspoons Dijon mustard

1/8 teaspoon ground red pepper

In a large bowl, combine bread crumbs, beef, turkey, mushrooms, onion, garlic, eggs, Italian seasoning, and salt. Mix well using your hands or a large spoon.

Spray a 9x6 loaf pan with cooking spray, place the meat loaf into the loaf pan. Place the loaf pan in the bottom of a large slow cooker.

In a medium bowl, whisk together ketchup, mustard, and pepper. Spread this mixture over the meat loaf, cover and cook on low for 5 to 6 hours or until meat loaf reaches 165 degrees F.

Allow the meat loaf to cook for about 20 minutes, then remove and slice.

CHEESE RAVIOLI

MEATS › CHEESE RAVIOLI, PASTA SAUCE, TOMATO SAUCE, ITALIAN SEASONING, MOZZARELLA

SERVES: 6

1 (25 ounces) bag of cheese ravioli

1 (26 ounces) jar pasta sauce

1 (8 ounces) can of tomato sauce

1 cup of water

2 teaspoons Italian seasoning

1 cup shredded mozzarella cheese

Pour half of the pasta sauce in the bottom of a large slow cooker. Add the frozen ravioli on top of the sauce. In a large bowl, combine the remaining pasta sauce, tomato sauce, Italian seasoning, and water. Mix well. Pour mixture over the frozen ravioli.

Cover and cook on low for 4 to 5 hours. About 15 minutes before serving, sprinkle with mozzarella cheese and allow to melt.

TARRAGON CHICKEN

MEATS › CHICKEN BREAST, TARRAGON, ONION, SALT, PEPPER

SERVES: 4

2 split chicken breasts

2 cups loosely packed fresh tarragon

1 onion, sliced

1/4 teaspoon salt

1/4 teaspoon freshly ground black pepper

Place the chicken in a 4-quart slow cooker. Top with remaining ingredients. Cook on low for 7–8 hours.

Remove the chicken from the slow cooker. Peel off the skin and discard. Discard the tarragon and onion.

PORK SHOULDER STUFFED WITH FENNEL, GARLIC, AND ROSEMARY

MEATS › PORK SHOULDER, GARLIC, ROSEMARY, FENNEL SEEDS, ONION, WHITE WHINE

SERVES: 8

One 5- to 6 pounds boneless pork shoulder

1 tablespoon sea salt

2 teaspoons freshly ground black pepper

1/2 cup extra-virgin olive oil

6 garlic cloves, minced

2 tablespoons finely chopped fresh rosemary

2 teaspoons fennel seeds

2 large onions, finely chopped

1 fennel bulb, wispy fronds removed, finely chopped

2 cups dry white wine, such as Pinot Grigio or Sauvignon Blanc, or dry vermouth

Lay the pork on a cutting board, fat-side down, and sprinkle with some of the salt and pepper. In a mixing bowl, stir together the remaining salt and pepper, olive oil, garlic, rosemary, and fennel seeds. Rub this mixture all over the pork. Roll up the pork from a short side, and tie it at 1 -in intervals with butcher's twine or silicone loops.

Spread out the onions and chopped fennel on the bottom of the insert for a 5- to 7-quart slow cooker, and pour in the wine. Lay the pork on t op of the vegetables. Cover and cook on high for 5 to 6 hours, or on low for 10 to 12 hours. The pork will be very tender. Remove the meat from the slow cooker, cover with aluminum foil, and allow to rest for 20 minutes.

Strain the contents of the slow cooker into a saucepan and skim off any excess fat. Bring the sauce to a boil and continue boiling until reduced by half. Cut off the butcher's twine, and remove any excess fat. Slice the meat 1/2 in thick, or pull apart with two forks.

Serve piled on a platter with the sauce on the side.

CHICKEN PICCATA

MEATS › CHICKEN BREAST, CANOLA OIL, LEMON JUICE, NONPAREIL CAPERS, CHICKEN STOCK

SERVES: 4

2 boneless, skinless thin-cut chicken breasts

1 cup flour

1 teaspoon canola oil

1/4 cup lemon juice

3 tablespoons nonpareil capers

3/4 cup Chicken Stock

Dredge both sides of the chicken breasts in the flour. Discard leftover flour.

Heat the oil in a nonstick pan. Quickly sear the chicken on each side.

Place the chicken, lemon juice, capers, and stock into a 4-quart slow cooker.

Cook on high for 3 hours or for 6 hours on low.

PORK ROAST WITH MUSHROOMS

MEATS › PORK LOIN ROAST, CREAM MUSHROOM SOUP, ONION SOUP MIX

SERVES: 8

32 ounces pork loin roast

1 can cream of mushroom soup, low fat and sodium

1 package of onion soup mix

1 cup water

Place the roast in the bottom of a large slow cooker. In a large bowl, whisk soup, soup mix, and water together. Pour soup mixture over the roast. Cover and cook on low for 8 to 10 hours.

JALAPEÑO CHICKEN

MEATS › CHICKEN THIGHS, PEPPERONI, JALAPENO PEPPERS, CREAM CHEESE, MOZZARELLA

SERVES: 6

6 boneless, skinless chicken thighs

12 slices of pepperoni, diced

1/2 cup sliced pickled jalapeño peppers

4 ounces cream cheese, softened

1 cup shredded mozzarella cheese

Use a 4-quart slow cooker. Place the chicken into the insert. Top with the pepperoni and jalapeños. Dot cubes of cream cheese on the top, and add the mozzarella. Cover, and cook on low for 6 hours.

CHICKEN BROCCOLI CASSEROLE

MEATS › CHICKEN BREASTS, CREAM CHEESE, CHICKEN BROTH, CHEDDAR, BROCCOLI

6 chicken breasts

8 ounces cream cheese

1 cup organic chicken broth

1 cup organic mayo

4 ounces cheddar cheese, shredded

4 ounces Provolone cheese, shredded

4 cups frozen broccoli, thawed and chopped

sea salt and freshly ground black pepper to taste

Place the chicken, cream cheese, broth and mayo in a slow cooker on low for 4-5 hours or until chicken is fork tender and cooked through.

Shred the chicken with a fork. Add the cheeses, broccoli and salt and pepper to taste.

Cook on low for an additional hour or until cheese is melted. Serve over Miracle Rice

GARLIC CHICKEN FOR 2

MEATS › CHICKEN BREAST, GARLIC, SALT, PEPPER

SERVES: 2

20 whole cloves of garlic

1 split chicken breast

1/8 teaspoon salt

1/8 teaspoon black pepper

Peel the garlic cloves. Sprinkle the chicken with salt and pepper.

Place the chicken breast and garlic cloves in a 1 1/2- to 2-quart slow cooker. Cook on low for 6–7 hours.

CREAMY MEXICAN CHICKEN

MEATS › CHICKEN BREAST, TOMATOES, SALSA, CREAM CHEESE

SERVES: 6

2 pounds uncooked frozen chicken breast

11/2 cups diced tomatoes

16 ounces salsa

8 ounces cream cheese

Place the frozen chicken breasts in a 4-quart slow cooker, top with tomatoes and salsa. Cook on low for 6 to 8 hours or until chicken is cooked.

Place block of cream cheese on top. Cook for an additional 30 minutes. Whisk to incorporate cream cheese into sauce. The stirring will cause the chicken to shred.

Serve on top of cauliflower rice or miracle rice.

BACON RANCH CHICKEN

MEATS › CHICKEN BREAST, CHICKEN SOUP, TURKEY BACON, CHICKEN BROTH, PEAS

SERVES: 4

4 boneless chicken breasts

1 can fat free, low sodium cream of chicken soup

6 slices turkey bacon, cooked and chopped

8 ounces fat free chicken broth

8 ounces package frozen peas

1 packet ranch dressing mix

In a medium bowl, mix soup, ranch dressing mix, and broth. Place chicken, peas, and bacon in the bottom of a large slow cooker. Pour soup mixture over chicken. Cover and cook on high for 4 hours. Serve over cauliflower rice or miracle rice.

TOMATO-BRAISED PORK

MEATS › PORK ROAST, CRUSHED TOMATOES, TOMATO PASTE, MARJORAM

SERVES: 4

28 ounces canned crushed tomatoes

3 tablespoons tomato paste

1 cup loosely packed fresh basil

1/2 teaspoon freshly ground black pepper

1/2 teaspoon marjoram

1 1/4 pounds boneless pork roast

1 packet ranch dressing mix

Place the tomatoes, tomato paste, basil, pepper, and marjoram into a 4-quart slow cooker. Stir to create a uniform sauce. Add the pork.

Cook on low for 7–8 hours or until the pork easily falls apart when poked with a fork.

Vegetarian

ARTICHOKE STUFFED MUSHROOMS

VEGETARIAN › BUTTON MUSHROOMS, ONION, GARLIC, ARTICHOKE, CREAM CHEESE, NUTMEG, PARMESAN

SERVES: 12

1 tablespoon coconut oil

1/4 cup onion, chopped

1 clove garlic, minced

24 button mushrooms, stems removed and chopped

1 (12-ounces) jar marinated artichoke hearts, drained and chopped

8 ounces cream cheese, softened

1 cup Asiago or Parmesan, finely shredded

1/4 teaspoon nutmeg

1/4 teaspoon sea salt and freshly ground black pepper

Heat the oil in a skillet over medium heat; cook the onions, garlic and mushroom stems in the hot oil until the onion is translucent, about 5 minutes; season with salt and pepper.

Transfer the mixture to a large bowl; add the artichoke hearts, cream cheese and Asiago. Season with nutmeg, salt and pepper. Stir the mixture until ingredients are evenly distributed.

Stuff the mushroom caps with the mixture. Arrange the stuffed mushrooms in a 4-quart or larger slow cooker.

Cook on high for 2 hours and serve warm.

BLACK BEAN AND TOMATO QUINOA

VEGETARIAN › BLACK BEANS, QUINOA, TOMATOES, CILANTRO, GARLIC, GREEN ONION, LIME

SERVES: 2-4

1 cup dried black beans, soaked overnight and drained

1 cup quinoa, rinsed

2 ripe tomatoes, diced

1/4 cup chopped fresh cilantro leaves

2 garlic cloves, chopped

4 green onions, thinly sliced

1 lime, juiced

2 cups vegetable or chicken broth

freshly grated Parmesan cheese, (optional)

Use a 4-quart slow cooker. Put the beans into the insert. Add the quinoa, tomatoes, cilantro, garlic, green onion, and lime juice. Stir in the broth.

Cover, and cook on low for 6 hours, or on high for 3 hours, until the beans have reached desired tenderness. Uncover and unplug the slow cooker. Fluff the quinoa with a fork, and let the pot sit for 10 minutes with the lid off to let condensation escape. Serve as is, or with a sprinkle of cheese, if desired.

SPICED EGGPLANT

VEGETARIAN › EGGPLANT, ONION, RED PEPPER FLAKES, ROSEMARY, LEMON

SERVES: 4

1 pound cubed eggplant

1/3 cup sliced onion

1/2 teaspoon red pepper flakes

1/2 teaspoon crushed rosemary

1/4 cup lemon juice

Place all ingredients in a 1 1/2–2-quart slow cooker. Cook on low for 3 hours or until the eggplant is tender.

VEGGIE CHILI

VEGETARIAN › CARROTS, CELERY, ONION, MUSHROOMS, ZUCCHINI, SQUASH, BASIL BEANS

SERVES: 15

1 cup carrots, chopped

1 cup celery, chopped

1 medium onion, chopped

16 ounces sliced fresh mushrooms, sliced

1 large zucchini, chopped

1 yellow squash, chopped

1 tablespoon chili powder

1 teaspoon seasoned pepper

1 teaspoon dried basil

24 ounces tomato juice

8 ounces can tomato sauce

2 (14 ounces) cans diced tomatoes, undrained

1 (15 ounces) can pinto beans, rinsed and drained

1 (15 ounces) can northern beans, rinsed and drained

1 (15 ounces) can black beans, rinsed and drained

1 (15 ounces) can red kidney beans, rinsed and drained

8 oz. frozen corn

Place all Ingredients into a large slow cooker and stir until well mixed. Cover and cook on low for 6 to 8 hours or until veggies are tender and the soup is thickened. Serve warm.

RATATOUILLE

VEGETARIAN › ONION, EGGPLANT, ZUCCHINI, CUBANELLE PEPPER, TOMATOES, BASIL, PARSLEY, TOMATO PASTE

SERVES: 4

1 onion, roughly chopped

1 eggplant, sliced horizontally

2 zucchini, sliced

1 cubanelle pepper, sliced

3 tomatoes, cut into wedges

2 tablespoons minced fresh basil

2 tablespoons minced fresh Italian parsley

1/4 teaspoon salt

1/2 teaspoon freshly ground black pepper

3 ounces tomato paste

1/4 cup water

Place the onion, eggplant, zucchini, pepper, and tomatoes into a 4-quart slow cooker. Sprinkle with basil, parsley, salt, and pepper.

Whisk the tomato paste and water in a small bowl. Pour the mixture over the vegetables. Stir.

Cook on low for 4 hours or until the eggplant and zucchini are fork-tender.

BUTTERY MUSHROOMS

VEGETARIAN › MUSHROOMS, BUTTER, MARJORAM, CHIVES, BROTH, RED WINE VINEGAR

SERVES: 8

1 pound mushrooms, quartered

1/2 cup butter or coconut oil

1 tablespoon marjoram

1 teaspoon chives, minced

1/2 cup organic veggie or chicken broth

2 tablespoon red wine vinegar

sea salt and freshly ground black pepper to taste

Clean and quarter mushrooms. Place mushrooms in a 2-quart slow cooker. Place the butter, marjoram, chives, broth and vinegar in the slow cooker. Season with salt and pepper.

Cover and cook for 4 hours on low or until soft

VEGGIE STEW

VEGETARIAN › GARLIC, CELERY, CARROTS, BUTTERNUT SQUASH, BUTTON MUSHROOMS, POTATOES, WHITE BEANS

SERVES: 6

3/4 cup vegetable broth

3 garlic cloves, minced

1 medium onion, chopped

1 cup celery, chopped

2 cups carrots, chopped

1 small butternut squash, peeled, deseeded, and largely diced

8 ounces button mushrooms, sliced

3 large white potatoes, peeled and diced

15 ounces can white beans

15 ounces can fire roasted crushed tomatoes

sea salt and freshly ground black pepper to taste

In a large slow cooker, layer garlic, onion, celery, carrots, squash, mushrooms, and potatoes. Pour the beans, broth, and tomatoes over the vegetables. Cover and cook on low for 6 hours or until vegetables are tender.

CREAMY FENNEL

VEGETARIAN › FENNEL BULBS, HEAVY CREAM, PARMESAN

SERVES: 4

2 large fennel bulbs, stalks removed, halved lengthwise, and cut in 1/2 inch wedges

1/2 cup heavy cream

1 cup finely grated Parmesan

sea salt and freshly ground black pepper to taste

Grease a 4-quart slow cooker. In a bowl, toss together fennel, cream, and 1 cup Parmesan; season with salt and pepper.

Cover and cook on low for 4-6 hours or until fennel is tender.

Sides

CREAMY CAULIFLOWER WITH BACON

SIDES › BACON, CHEDDAR, CAULIFLOWER, PARSLEY

SERVES: 8-10

vegetable oil spray

4 ounces bacon (about 4 slices), minced

1 (11-ounce) can condensed cheddar cheese soup

1/4 cup water

sea salt and freshly ground black pepper

2 cups shredded cheddar cheese (8 ounces)

2 heads cauliflower (4 pounds), cored, 1 head cut into 1-inch florets (6 cups), 1 head chopped coarse (6 cups)

1 tablespoon minced fresh parsley

Line slow cooker with aluminum foil collar and coat with vegetable oil spray. Cook bacon in large pot over medium heat until crisp, 5 to 7 minutes. Transfer bacon to paper towel–lined plate and refrigerate until serving. Pour off all bacon fat left in pot.

Bring condensed soup, water, 1/2 teaspoon pepper, and 1/2 teaspoon salt to simmer in pot. Slowly whisk in 1 1/2 cups cheddar until completely melted; stir in cauliflower and coat evenly with sauce.

Transfer cauliflower mixture to prepared slow cooker and sprinkle with remaining 1/2 cup cheddar. Cover and cook until cauliflower is tender, 4 to 6 hours on low.

Remove foil collar, stir cauliflower well, and season with salt and pepper to taste. Microwave bacon on paper towel–lined plate until hot and crisp, about 30 seconds. Sprinkle cauliflower with crisp bacon and parsley before serving.

WILD RICE WITH MIXED VEGETABLES

SIDES › WILD RICE, CLOVES, ONION, CARROT, CELERY

SERVES: 8

2 1/2 cups water

1 cup wild rice

3 cloves garlic, minced

1 medium onion, diced

1 carrot, diced

1 stalk celery, diced

Place all ingredients into a 4-quart slow cooker and stir. Cover and cook on low for 4 hours. After 4 hours, check to see if the kernels are open and tender. If not, put the lid back on, and continue to cook for an additional 15–30 minutes. Stir before serving.

GREEK MUSHROOMS

SIDES › MUSHROOMS, BUTTER, GARLIC, LAMB, PAPRIKA, PARSLEY, FETA

SERVES: 20

20 large mushrooms

2 tablespoons butter or coconut oil

1/2 medium red onion, diced

2 cloves garlic, minced

1/2 pounds ground lamb or sausage

1 teaspoon sea salt

1/2 teaspoon ground black pepper

1/2 teaspoon paprika

1/4 cup fresh parsley, chopped

4 ounces feta cheese, crumbled

Wash the mushrooms, remove the stems. Set caps aside on a paper towel to dry. Finely chop stems.

In a skillet over medium heat, add the oil, onion, garlic and mushroom stems. Cook 2-3 minutes until onion begins to soften. Add the lamb or sausage. Season with salt, pepper, and paprika and cook until lightly browned through.

Transfer the sausage to a mixing bowl along with the parsley and feta cheese.

Stir to combine ingredients and stuff 1 tablespoon of mixture in each cap.

Place mushrooms in the slow cooker. Cover. Cook on High for 2 hours.

BACON CHEESE MUSHROOMS

SIDES › PORTOBELLO MUSHROOMS, BACON, GARLIC, CREAM CHEESE, CHEDDAR

SERVES: 12

16 ounces portobello mushrooms

8 ounces bacon

1/2 cup onion, minced

1 clove garlic, minced

4 ounces cream cheese

1/4 cup grated sharp cheddar cheese

sea salt and freshly ground black pepper

Remove mushroom stems from caps and chop stems in small pieces.

Chop the bacon in small pieces. In a large sauté pan, over medium heat, cook bacon, onion, garlic and chopped mushroom stems until the bacon is crispy. Reduce heat to low. Add cream cheese and cheddar cheese in the sauté pan and stir until cheeses are melted. Season with salt and pepper.

Remove mixture from heat and stuff each mushroom cap generously with mixture.

Place the mushrooms in a 4-quart slow cooker on high for 1 hour or on low for 2 hours. Serve warm from slow cooker.

MASHED SWEET POTATOES

SIDES › SWEET POTATOES, BUTTER, HEAVY CREAM, SUGAR

SERVES: 6

3 pounds sweet potatoes (about 4 medium), peeled and cut into 1-inch chunks

1 1/2 cups water

sea salt and freshly ground black pepper

6 tablespoons unsalted butter, melted

3 tablespoons heavy cream, warmed, plus extra as needed

1 1/2 teaspoons sugar

Combine potatoes, water, and 1 teaspoon salt in slow cooker. Cover and cook until potatoes are tender, 4 to 6 hours on low.

Drain potatoes, then return to slow cooker. Mash potatoes thoroughly with potato masher. Fold in butter, cream, and sugar. Add more cream as needed to adjust consistency. Season with salt and pepper to taste and serve.

RED BEANS AND RICE

SIDES › ONION, GARLIC, CELERY, BEANS, TOMATOES, CHILE, OREGANO, PAPRIKA, THYME, RICE

SERVES: 8

1 teaspoon canola oil

1 small onion, diced

3 cloves garlic, minced

1 stalk celery, diced

15 ounces canned kidney beans, drained and rinsed

15 ounces canned diced tomatoes

4 ounces canned green chile

1/2 teaspoon dried oregano

1/2 teaspoon hot paprika

1/2 teaspoon cayenne pepper

1/2 teaspoon dried thyme

2 cups cooked long-grain rice

Heat the canola oil in a nonstick pan. Sauté the onions, garlic, and celery until the onions are soft, about 5 minutes.

Add the onion mixture, beans, tomatoes, chiles, and spices to a 1 1/2- to 2-quart slow cooker. Cook on low for 6–8 hours. Remove the contents to a large bowl and stir in the rice.

Desserts

CHOCOLATE MOUSSE

DESSERTS › EGGS, WHIPPING CREAM, ESPRESSO, VANILLA, CHOCOLATE

SERVES: 8

2 cups heavy whipping cream

4 large egg yolks

1 1/4 cup Swerve, Confectioners (or equivalent)

1/3 cup espresso or strong coffee

1 teaspoon vanilla extract

1 cup unsweetened baking chocolate, chopped fine

In a 4-quart slow cooker (if you use larger, it will cook faster), place the heavy cream, yolks, natural sweetener, espresso and extract. Whisk until combined. Add the chocolate.

Cover and cook on low for about two hours.

Once the chocolate is melted and there are little bubbles on top, carefully pour the mixture in a blender. Blend on high until it "grows" to almost double in size. Pour into serving dishes and chill for 2 hours or overnight in the refrigerator. Top with whipped cream if desired.

CHEESECAKE

DESSERTS › LOW FAT CHOCOLATE, CREAM CHEESE, SUGAR, EGG, VANILLA, FLOUR, LEMON

SERVES: 8

3/4 cup low-fat chocolate or cinnamon graham cracker crumbs

1 1/2 tablespoons butter, melted

8 ounces reduced-fat sour cream, at room temperature

8 ounces reduced-fat cream cheese, at room temperature

2/3 cup sugar

1 egg, at room temperature

1 tablespoon vanilla paste or vanilla extract

1 1/2 tablespoons flour

1 tablespoon lemon juice

1 tablespoon lemon zest

In a small bowl, mix together the graham cracker crumbs and butter. Press into the bottom and sides of a 6 inches springform pan.

In a large bowl, mix the sour cream, cream cheese, sugar, egg, vanilla, flour, lemon juice, and zest until completely smooth. Pour into the springform pan.

Pour 1 inch of water into the bottom of a 6-quart slow cooker. Place a trivet in the bottom of the slow cooker. Place the pan onto the trivet.

Cook on low for 2 hours. Turn off the slow cooker and let the cheesecake steam for 1 hour and 15 minutes with the lid on. Remove the cheesecake from the slow cooker. Refrigerate 6 hours or overnight before serving.

TROPICAL BANANAS FOSTER

DESSERTS › BROWN SUGAR, BUTTER, COCONUT MILK, DARK RUM, PINEAPPLE, CINNAMON, BANANAS, VANILLA ICE CREAM

SERVES: 8

cooking spray

1/2 cup packed dark brown sugar

3 tablespoons butter

1/4 cup light coconut milk

1/4 cup dark rum

1 cup (1-inch) cubed fresh pineapple

1/4 teaspoon ground cinnamon

4 ripe bananas, cut into 1/2-inch-thick slices

1 3/4 cups vanilla light ice cream

Coat a 3-quart electric slow cooker with cooking spray. Combine brown sugar and next 3 ingredients (through rum) in slow cooker. Cover and cook on low for 1 hour. Stir with a whisk until smooth.

Add pineapple, cinnamon, and banana to sauce, stirring to coat. Cover and cook on low for 15 minutes. Serve immediately over ice cream.

CINNAMON APPLES

DESSERTS › APPLES, LEMON, BROWN SUGAR, WALNUTS, MAPLE SYRUP, BUTTER, DRIED CRANBERRIES, CINNAMON

SERVES: 6

6 medium Granny Smith apples, peeled and cut into eighths

1 tablespoon lemon juice

1/2 cup firmly packed dark brown sugar

1/2 cup chopped walnuts

1/2 cup maple syrup

1/4 cup sweetened dried cranberries

1/4 cup butter, melted

2 teaspoons ground cinnamon

2 tablespoons water

1 tablespoon cornstarch

Combine apples and lemon juice in a 4-quart slow cooker; toss well to coat. Add brown sugar and next 5 ingredients, combining well.

Cover and cook on low 3 hours.

Stir together water and cornstarch in a small bowl; stir into apples.

Cover and cook on low 3 more hours or until apples are tender.

SLOW COOKED PINEAPPLE

DESSERTS › PINEAPPLE, VANILLA BEAN, RUM

SERVES: 8

1 whole pineapple, peeled

1 vanilla bean, split

3 tablespoons water or rum

Place all ingredients into a 4-quart oval slow cooker. Cook on low for 4 hours or until fork tender. Remove the vanilla bean before serving.

1/8 teaspoon	0.5 milliliter
1/4 teaspoon	1 milliliter
1/2 teaspoon	2 milliliters
1 teaspoon	5 milliliters
1/2 tablespoon	7 milliliters

1 tablespoon (3 teaspoons)	15 milliliters
2 tablespoons (1 fluid ounce)	30 milliliters
1 / 4 cup (4 tablespoons)	60 milliliters
1 / 3 cup	90 milliliters
1 / 2 cup (4 fluid ounces)	125 milliliters
2 / 3 cup	160 milliliters
3 / 4 cup (6 fluid ounces)	180 milliliters

1 cup (16 tablespoons)	250 milliliters
1 pint (2 cups)	500 milliliters
1 quart (4 cups)	1 liter (about)
1/2 ounce	15 grams
1 ounce	30 grams
2 ounces	60 grams

3 ounces	85 grams
1 / 4 pound (4 ounces)	115 grams
1 / 2 pound (8 ounces)	225 grams
3 / 4 pound (12 ounces)	340 grams
1 pound (16 ounces)	454 grams

200 degrees F	95 degrees C
250 degrees F	120 degrees C
275 degrees F	135 degrees C
300 degrees F	150 degrees C
325 degrees F	160 degrees C
350 degrees F	180 degrees C
375 degrees F	190 degrees C
400 degrees F	205 degrees C

| 425 degrees F | 220 degrees C |
| 450 degrees F | 230 degrees C |

9 781999 283254